Porn Addiction Recovered: The Ultimate Guide to Stop Porn Obsessing: Science of Pornography Addiction Revealed

I0421474

Check Out My Other Books

Sex Addiction Recovered: The Ultimate Guide to Stop Sex Obsessing: Science of Sex Addiction Revealed

Table of Contents

Part I
Getting Started

Introduction

I want to thank you and congratulate you for downloading the book, *Porn Addiction Recovered: The Ultimate Guide to Stop Porn Obsessing: Science of Pornography Addiction Revealed.*

Porn Addiction Recovered is your one-stop source for obtaining tools based on research that will allow you to better understand pornography addiction, how to recover from the addiction, and how to maintain recovery. There is hope to become and stay free.

Topics include:

What is Porn Addiction?

The Consequences

Cybersex

The Addiction Cycle

Porn Addiction and the Brain

Family Dynamics

Breaking Free from Porn Addiction with Evidence-Based Tools

Healthy Sex Maintenance

Relapse Prevention

And more...

Porn Addiction Recovered is the ultimate guide to achieve the quality of life you deserve and break the porn addiction cycle for good.

This is a book for those who have longed to break the porn addiction cycle as well as for those who are in relationships with individuals struggling with porn addiction. This book is based on evidence and is written by a health psychology professional.

This book is not just about breaking the porn addiction cycle. By learning to work through the causes and utilize evidence-based tools, you will feel more centered, more confident, more joyous, and cope better with emotions and life's stressors. There are endless possibilities when you finally break free from porn addiction.

Celebrate the joy of breaking free from porn addiction and maintaining healthy intimacy with *Porn Addiction Recovered*.

Chapter One

What is Porn Addiction?

Pornography addiction is very similar to other addictions. It is not just a habit, but has compulsive components. People who use porn excessively often feel as if they have uncontrollable cravings and urges. Porn addiction affects people of all ages, ethnic backgrounds, religions, and of all cultural backgrounds. Porn addiction is a form of compulsive sexual behavior.

Porn addiction falls under the category of sex addiction as it is a sexual compulsivity issue. The word "porn" is typed into about a quarter of a million internet searches per day. There are over a billion websites worldwide of internet porn. Up to 8 percent of Americans are addicted to sex. Seventy percent of sex addicts report having a problem with online sexual behavior.

Porn addiction can be defined as a behavioral addiction (like gambling or binge eating) that is characterized by an ever-growing compulsion or need to view pornographic content or material. In the past, a person suffering from an addiction to porn would satisfy his/her craving for porn content by viewing or storing explicit videos, magazines and photos. The tools available to feed a porn addiction have since evolved along with technology, by providing unlimited pornography at all levels of explicitness. Additionally, today's porn addiction is also enabled by a range of devices such as the social media, apps, virtual reality technology, and phones. These devices are enabling for a porn addict because they allow a person to store and view porn in higher volumes than ever before while leaving little or no trace of use.

Millions of Americans struggle with porn addiction for years in secret and continue their porn-seeking behavior even after it begins to have negative consequences in their lives.

For some individuals, images are enough. For others, porn is a gateway to compulsive and risky sexual behavior with others.

Warning Signs that there may be a problem:

- If you are distressed by the behavior
- If the pornography used is interfering with work, finances, relationships or any other major area of functioning in life
- If the partner is distressed by the behavior
- If you have tried to stop and failed

Common signs that casual porn use has escalated to the level of addiction include:

- Continued porn use despite consequences and/or promises to stop
- Increasing the amount of time spent on porn use
- Significant periods of time (hours or days) lost to finding and viewing pornography
- Needing to increase the intensity or type of sexual content viewed in order to get a fix
- Lying and covering up the nature and extent of porn use
- Using porn to escape negative emotions such as sadness, boredom, stress, or anger
- Anger or irritability if asked to stop

- Loss of interest in sexual relationships with spouses or partners
- Not being present in relationships or disconnecting from others
- Using drugs or alcohol in conjunction with porn
- Objectifying men or women, or viewing them as body parts rather than people
- Escalation to using the Internet for anonymous sexual hookups or to find prostitutes

If someone uses pornography on a regular basis, however, they do not feel distressed by it, and they do not exhibit any of the formerly noted warning signs, clinical professionals would not identify the pornography use as problem behavior.

The biggest problem with porn use is that there is a physiologically addictive nature to porn and all sexually addictive behavior. People build up a tolerance and need more and more stimulation to achieve the same high. Therefore, someone might start by looking at images of an adult couple having sex and then move on to watching bestiality or sex with children. Twenty percent off all Internet porn involves children, according to a 2003 study. People push their edge in order to obtain a better high and a better distraction from life's stressors.

Online porn is so much about the hunt, which is part of why people spend so many hours at it, at the expense of their jobs, family, social life and sleep. They continue searching for the image or video that is going to produce a high. It's similar to the drug addict going out to score the drug. However, there are many people who would never go to a prostitute who engage in online porn.

The availability of Internet porn has increased the prevalence of sex addiction behaviors, especially in young people. Fifteen or twenty years ago, a young boy might be thrilled to get his hands on a copy of a nude magazine to stare at photos of naked women. However, nowadays, male and female children and adolescents can watch videos on the internet of people actually having sex, some of it violent. Allowing your children access to internet porn is like allowing your children to play with crystal meth. For this reason, parental controls on their computers are advised. The danger of being exposed to porn early on is that it creates a distorted view of what sex is and its place in a relationship.

A significant worry for some is the risk for adolescents developing a porn addiction. If a person is exposed to pornography and they do not have a solid understanding of intimacy (of what love truly is) there can be difficulty. Until the age of twenty-one, a person's brain is not fully developed. Therefore, there is a chance for significant emotional and psychological disruption for children, adolescents, and young adults to be exposed to pornography.

Parents often want to ignore this topic. As difficult as those dialogues can be, sex therapists recommend the topic be discussed so that the child understands the difference between what they may see on a screen or magazine and what true intimacy looks like. They must understand that the sex depicted in pornography is "Hollywood" and not realistic.

Causes of Sex Addiction:

One of the causes of sex addiction can be neurochemical in nature given the fact that research has shown that antidepressants have been effective in sex addicts. All disorders are caused by a combination of genetics and environmental variables so it is assumed that environment and genetic predispositions play a role in the cause of sex addiction.

The reward center of the brain communicates that sex is necessary for survival. In sex addicts, the prefrontal cortex (the reasonable part of our brain that makes good decisions) becomes short-circuited and they become more likely to act on impulses. However, with treatment this can be reversed.

During acting out behaviors, a person will experience a sense of euphoria. The sex addict is usually seeking pleasure or relief to avoid challenging situations and distract from difficult emotions. Their actions typically result in feelings of shame, guilt, and remorse.

Eighty percent of recovering sex addicts report having some type of addiction in their families (such as binge eating, substance abuse or gambling). Sex addiction is an intimacy disorder. Sex addicts are seeking intimacy and instead of finding intimacy, they are putting other clinging to behaviors that will give them a false sense of intimacy. Sex addicts substitute intimacy for intensity. They may seek out experience that will give them physical pain or pleasure. They may also seek domination or submission type of experiences. Sex addiction is not defined by a particular behavior. People who have an affair or even more than one affair could or could not be sex addicted. A person who looks at pornography may be a sex addict or may not.

Many porn addicts disclose that they discovered porn early on in childhood. They typically did not know how to register that information and began to use it as a way to cope. Finding pornography in your parents' room or friend's house as a child can be a significant causal factor in porn addiction. Moreover, hardcore pornography can have a tremendous impact on the psyche.

Psychological abuse, physical abuse, and/or sexual abuse can be a significant causal factor of porn addiction. Additionally, those who were raised in strict religious homes can be more likely to develop a porn addiction due to the shame placed on them for masturbating or acting out sexually in any way. The more the fundamental (black and white/all or nothing/good and bad) the religious beliefs are, the more it has the potential for being a causal factor for porn addiction. Being raised with the idea that there is something is wrong with sex or the belief that sex/porn is something "We don't talk about" can be contributing factor in porn addiction.

Porn addicts are not likely to say no when they are deep into their addiction. They may have online sexual encounters, real-life encounters, or they may strictly view porn and watch it compulsively. The need for porn consumption can be so great that they don't know how to stop. Unfortunately, the pursuit of online sex and excessive porn can have life-changing consequences.

Porn addiction is using porn (thoughts about porn or porn-seeking behaviors) as an escape from uncomfortable feelings. Porn addicts often feel fearful, lonely, guilty, and, ashamed, and lost. However, the only way a porn addict knows to get over these difficult feelings is to return to the behavior that's also causing these negative emotions. Dopamine, serotonin, and adrenaline (feel-good chemicals in the brain) allow you to escape feelings that you want to avoid because of the high (at least for the short-term). When a porn addict feels there are no outlets for their sexual acting out they may feel restless, anxious, and even depressed.

There is a correlation between molestation (sex abuse) during childhood and porn addiction. Porn addicts often experience shame around the abuse and there is shame around the behaviors that come with porn addiction. Oftentimes, individuals who had been abused as children want to take back emotional power and control by acting out sexually.

Eighty-two percent of sex addicts (porn addiction is a form of sex addiction) have been sexually abused. When you're sexually abused, you are used as an object so you begin to connect sex to an object relationship instead of a personal or intimate relationship. Therefore, most sex addicts are medicating psychological pain. Many times, sex addicts describe their families as rigid, uncaring, and distant. Sex addicts typically come from dysfunctional families. Some sex addicts assert that they only felt loved as children when they were performing (doing something the authoritative figures demanded of them). As a result, the core belief of a sex addict is often "I am unlovable" or "I am loved only when I perform."

Scenarios of porn addiction:

- A 40-year-old married attorney views online pornography for hours at home, masturbating six to seven times a day, then begins surfing porn sites at the office and risks destroying his career.

- A woman spends four to seven hours a day in internet chat rooms and having cybersex, and eventually begins arranging to meet online strangers for casual sex in real life.

- A 20-year old man spends numerous hours a day downloading porn, filling multiple hard drives, and devotes a separate computer just to pornography. He turns down going to see friends and family constantly to the point where they no longer call.

Why do some people become compulsive with pornography?

Most people do not have a compulsion with pornography. However, there is a part of the population that is challenged with it. Some porn addicts have poor social skills. Some porn addicts have ADHD and that can be a contributor to excessive porn use. Studies show that individuals with ADHD are more vulnerable to excessive porn use. High sex drive can also make people more vulnerable to compulsive sexual behavior. Sometimes, when a couple's intimate relationship is not a good place (they feel distant, poor communication etc.) a person may use porn to replace intimacy. Porn addicts replace intimacy for *intensity*. However, it should be noted that even if there is poor communication or the addict feels disconnected, it is not the fault of the spouse or partner if porn is being used excessively by the addict.

Some porn addicts cannot talk about his or her feelings. If there are no outlets in place, a person may use porn to disconnect from feelings.

Porn addiction is not defined by what type of porn a person watches, what they are doing while watching porn, or even how often they are watching porn. Clinicians do not qualify addiction by how much you are engaging in porn addiction. However, clinicians do define porn use as an addiction if it is impairing your functioning in life (i.e. relationship problems, work problems, time with others lost, legal problems etc.).

Chapter Two

The Consequences and Realization

Porn addiction is a gigantic problem because people lose jobs over it. In 2008, Nielsen Online reported that 1/4 of employees use the internet to visit porn sites during the workday. Online porn sites report that highest usage is between the hours of 9 a.m. and 5 p.m. Numerous divorce attorneys report that pornography is a large issue in divorce at present, which it never was before the advent of the internet.

One major consequence of pornography abuse or addiction is the fact of desensitization. A person may start off watching porn that is relatively soft-core pornography and all of a sudden you may need something more intense like hard core pornography and more extreme genres (i.e. gang bang porn, physical abuse porn, rape porn, etc.). Long-term a person using porn excessively will require more and more and higher intensity porn in order to get the same feel-good chemicals to release in the brain.

Long-term effects of excessive porn use include an exaggerated perception of sexual activity of society, diminished trust between intimate couples, the abandonment of hope of sexual monogamy, and the belief that promiscuity is the natural state.

Other long-term negative effects of excessive porn use include:

- Voyeurism (an obsession of looking at people rather than interacting with them)
- Objectification (an attitude in which all people with whom you are attracted are objects by size, shape, body parts)
- Validation (the need to validate masculinity through beautiful women)
- Trophyism (the idea that beautiful people are collectible)
- Fear of true intimacy (inability to related to person you are attracted to in an honest and intimate way)
- Deep Loneliness-Some individuals will replace intimacy with intensity. This means the motivation can be lost to go out and find a partner. Porn addicts often isolate in their addiction and they do not reach out to others when they experience problems.
- Anger and Violence-Some individuals who use porn excessively report that porn brought them more anger and violence into their life that was not previously there.
- Erectile Dysfunctions-Men who use porn excessively, attribute arousal to watching a girl on a screen. When a man attempts to have sex with a woman in real life, it is not uncommon for a man to be unable to become erect. It can take months of abstaining from porn to return to normal sexual functioning.
- De-Valuation of Self-According to porn, you must have a large penis, large breasts, and a tight body to be valued. Porn can have a significant negative impact on self-image as well as confidence in the bedroom due to the

comparisons that we make when we watch porn. Porn has a paralyzing effect because it teaches us that you are solely valued in sex by having a large penis of you are a man or large breasts if you are a woman. Women get the notion that if they want to be valued they must be valued sexually.

- Shame Spiraling-shame can eat away at you. Shame can eat away at your self-esteem. It can diminish social confidence.
- Putting Sex on a Pedestal-Porn can make sex seem like a fantasy. Seeing sex as a fantasy-valuing large breasts and staged lighting instead of real touch of a person etc.
- Limiting Beliefs about Self-While they can make it harder to enjoy the actual act of sex, it can make you set limiting beliefs such as you are not worthy of having a real person have sex with you.

Many people who use porn excessively experience denial at some point. They can lie to themselves and others about how porn is negatively affecting their lives. It is important to keep in mind all of the reasons why porn is making your life worse can often help in deterring you from excessive usage. The reasons why you interpret porn as being unhealthy will depend on you, of course. Common reasons to not use porn include the negative impact it has on your spouse or family (what if you accidentally expose your kids or younger siblings?), the negative effect it has on your work, and the amount of time it sucks from your life. Define why exactly it is that you are driven to move away from excessive porn use so that it is solid in your mind for motivational purposes. On the following worksheet fill out the pros and cons of stopping and continuing the behavior. Then complete the worksheet called "Need for Change Assessment."

Decisions for Change Worksheet

Thinking through the pros and cons of making this change (as well as if you don't make the change) is a way to help you ensure that you have fully processed the prospect of the change.

Making a Change

Pros/Benefits

Cons/Costs

Not Changing

Pros/Benefits

Cons/Costs

Need for Change Assessment

Think about something you need or want to change related to sexual behaviors. Ask yourself the following questions.

Why do I want to make the change?

_____
_____
_____
_____
_____
_____
_____
_____

How will I make the change?

_____
_____
_____
_____
_____
_____
_____
_____
_____
_____
_____
_____
_____

What are some reasons to change?

_____
_____
_____
_____
_____
_____
_____
_____
_____
_____
_____
_____
_____
_____

What is your *ideal* outcome after making this change?

_____

_____

_____

_____

_____

_____

_____

_____

_____

_____

_____

_____

_____

_____

_____

_____

_____

_____

_____

_____

_____

Chapter Three

Cybersex

In 1980, the portion of the population who were sex addicted was 3.5 percent. Since the advent of the internet, however, the percentage has increased to 8 percent of the population. Cybersex is the access of any sexual content or experience through the internet. It has only been existence since the early 1990's. Cybersex is accessing any sex through the internet. It is important to note that not everyone with a sex addiction watches porn compulsively and not everyone who watches porn compulsively enters chat rooms or has cybersex. However, I have provided information on the subject for readers to understand cybersex from a psychological perspective.

For ninety percent of men, images are a big source of stimulation. Whereas women (an estimated twenty-five to thirty percent of online porn users) typically prefer interactive chat rooms. There are webcams with live men and women that are willing to interact with them. More than seventy percent of men age 18 to 34 visit a porn site in a time span of a month.

The anonymity of the internet allows a person to connect with others in chat rooms or online reality games without fear or insecurity, creating an image of oneself or an avatar that may bear little resemblance to who the person is in the real world. It is particularly difficult for porn addicts to stay away from internet porn because we are always on our computers, and it's always available. However, just like binge eaters who need to eat to survive and are surrounded by food, there is hope for recovery.

With the advent of internet, porn addiction is one of the fastest growing behavioral addictions. Many feel anxious if they are habituated to accessing porn or internet chat rooms. Many will miss important meetings to stay on the internet surfing porn. They may stay up late to watch porn or get onto internet chat rooms. Some people find that chat rooms are a way to connect in a "safe" way where a person does not have to be fully vulnerable. As a result, a person is unable to form an emotional connection because of replacing intimacy with intensity.

Some individuals move on from watching porn to visiting chat rooms. Virtual reality sex is now a reality. It will become as mainstream as porn making it even more intense and difficult to stop. People may prefer to have digital sexuality as a result of avatars and a virtual sex. This involves putting on goggles and entering online communities to engage. Those who are attracted to these types of sexual encounters are typically avoiding real intimacy.

At times, excessive porn use can lead to escalated behaviors when one forms a tolerance to porn. One of these behaviors is engaging in cybersex. Cybersex is online sex or having sex on the internet. Cybersex is available on your phone or laptop. It is something that most people keep secret. Cybersex can temporarily fill the need for porn addicts to obtain a high that they used to be able to obtain simply from watching porn. Cybersex can be highly addictive just as porn addiction and it is an escalation from porn use alone.

There are three main criteria that indicate whether a person's engagement in cybersex is a problem:

Loss of control- you tell yourself or partner you are not going to do a behavior and you find yourself doing it again and again.

Consequences are happening in the person's life-you've lost a job, someone has left you, your children walked in and found you looking at porn etc.

Obsessive Thinking-A persons spends a great deal of time thinking about the behavior. Preoccupation and obsession of sex or porn is taking over your mind.

The most pleasure we can experienced without drugs is with sex. When someone has endless access to sexual experiences and content, and they can hide it very easily, it is so much easier for people to lose themselves in that experience. Unfortunately, individuals will never run out of porn because of the internet. The anticipation as well as the act of engaging in cybersex release feel-good chemicals and they are not aware of what is going on around them. However, when someone is addicted to cybersex, sex, or porn, they have tunnel vision and hyper-focus on the sexual experience. They are caught up in a loop of sexual arousal and excitement. As long as a person can maintain the sensory excitement, the person can distract from the fact that a boss yelled at them earlier, their memory of abuse was triggered, or they are stressed about money.

It is important to ask yourself how much time you spend on cybersex. It is also important to ask yourself how this is affecting your partner. Also, ask yourself what you are losing as a result of engaging in cybersex (i.e. time with children, friends, work production etc.). Individuals, couples, families, and careers can be destroyed when someone becomes out of control with porn or online sex. Overall, sex addiction is an emotional disorder that needs to be treated with care and compassion so that recovery can begin.

Part II
Inside the Addiction

Chapter Four

The Addiction Cycle and Shame

A person is not a sex addict or a porn addict simply because he/she watches porn. In order to have an addiction, the behavior must be interfering with a major area of functioning in a person's life.

What are the things that bring us pleasure? Community, eating, exercise, sexuality etc. Nature already rewards us for the things we need to survive. The problems is that for certain people who have really profound kinds of trauma and abuse in the family, mental health problems, and neglect they can be more susceptible to porn addiction. They may not have been able to form a deep sense of trust early on when it comes to deep intimacy in sexuality so they are handicapped when it comes to being vulnerable and intimate. They are often hunting fantasy and sexuality in order to escape emotional pain. They are a lot like compulsive gamblers. They are looking for the better game; they can't wait to cash their check; time goes by; and they run out of money. They lose themselves in the excitement of gaming and gambling just like porn addicts lose themselves in excessive porn use.

The Addiction Cycle

Preoccupation

Preoccupation involves thinking about the behavior (thinking about when you are going to have time to go to watch porn; fantasizing about the acting out behavior etc.). This preoccupation can last for hours or days.

Ritualization

The ritual falls between the preoccupation and the acting out phases. Ritualization is anything one does between thinking about the behavior and acting out on the behavior. It is essentially the stage in which someone is ruminating and preparing for the act. Waiting to be alone or turning on the computer is a type of ritual. Rituals from various addictions can overlap with each other. Drinking or eating could be part of the ritual leading up to the behavior. Rituals can be short or long.

A large part of a ritual is the thought process. What are you doing in your mind that is justifying the behaviors to yourself? Conversations with yourself allow you to attempt to justify the porn addict behaviors. If a person is engaged in the ritual, it most often leads to the acting out behavior.

As people move closer to the actual acting out they engage in a ritual. It prepares the body to the final culmination of acting out (in this case masturbating to porn for hours on end). It becomes much harder to turn back once a person is in the ritualization stage.

Compulsive Behavior (Acting out)

The Compulsive Behavior stage is when the acting out behavior is occurring. It is the stage in which the problematic behavior is present. This could be downloading porn, streaming porn, entering chat rooms for online sex etc.

Despair

Feelings of guilt and shame are characterized by the fourth phase of the sex addiction cycle. After acting out, the feeling of shame and guilt is the crash. These feelings trigger the cycle to begin over again. Most people with sex addiction feel badly after acting out on the behavior.

Sex addiction (for which porn addiction falls under) is not fun. Sex addiction is about looking for something outside of yourself to make yourself feel better. If a person has a bad day, he/she typically seeks a calming experience. With sex/porn addicts, they don't turn to calming soothing experiences to make themselves feel better. They seek intensity to avoid negative emotions. They also do not trust so they will isolate instead of connecting to others which is the exact opposite of a healthy way to cope. Porn addicts don't want to turn to others because they worry that they won't be soothed and may be let down. They feel that they can rely and depend on the distraction that porn provides.

Internet images never end. Cybersex is easily accessible which makes it extremely difficult to avoid. However, there are safety precautions one can pursue such as setting parental controls on your own computer, turning your computer to face the door, rearranging your work space so that it does not remind you as much of the old behavior.

Secrets and lying are what will ultimately hurt the relationship when it comes to cybersex. If someone says to their partner that they don't do anything sexual online and the partner finds it they will feel betrayed. The spouse or partner sees the discovery as devastating.

Chapter Five

Porn Addiction and the Brain

At Cambridge, they did a study of 19 porn addicted men compared to non-porn users. A neuropsychiatrist found greater activity in the area of the brain called ventral striatum (the reward center of the brain) which is a section of the brain that lights up when feel-good neurochemicals such as dopamine.

The reward center of the brain communicates that sex is necessary for survival. In sex addicts, the prefrontal cortex (the reasonable part of our brain that makes good decisions) becomes short-circuited and they become more likely to act on impulses. However, with treatment this can be reversed.

During sexual acting out behaviors, a person will experience a sense of euphoria. The addict is typically seeking pleasure or relief to avoid difficult situations and distract from negative emotions. Their actions typically result in guilt, shame, and remorse.

Porn addicts often feel as if they have uncontrollable urges. They are strong because they come from the limbic system. It is the part of the brain that is denser than other brain structures and it evolved before rational thought. This explains why urges are incredibly strong and it also explains why avoiding the behavior can actually feed the craving. Cravings and urges originate in the primal part of the brain. For some, porn has become such a regular part of their life-just like eating. If addiction is threatened, they experience a fight or flight response. Most people, when considering quitting an addictive behavior, experience a great deal of fear and anxiety around being without the drug to relieve tension or stress.

Sex addicts are most likely reenacting arousal patterns from their early childhood trauma, which in turn, further solidifies those patterns in the brain. The trauma could have been physical, emotional, or sexual abuse. Emotional trauma could look like a mother that was ill and emotionally unavailable. Physical abuse could have been a father coming home from work and punishing by pushing children around. Sexual abuse could have taken place during one incident or for a duration of many years.

The actual act of being close to something that you are watching works directly with the seeking pathway within the brain and it's the seeking pathway where dopamine is produced. When we experience dopamine release, we experience feelings of pleasure and satisfaction. Dopamine also motivates to try and seek more of it. The more dopamine you produce, the more your brain wants, so you find yourself wanting more and more of a substance or behavior to get that same high. What gets reinforced will get repeated. This can be for the good (i.e. exercise) and for the challenging (i.e. excessive porn use).

A trigger is something that reminds the addict of the behavior. Sexual triggers occur when the brain registers something through sight, scent, taste, sound, etc. This could be a sex scene in a movie, a billboard advertisement, or a radio show that has sexual undertones or overtones. Non-sexual environmental triggers also exist. An example of a non-sexual environmental trigger could be driving by a street because that is the one that led you to the sex store that has the porn you used to consume. The street is non-sexual yet it triggers you. A room in your house or an empty house could also be examples of non-sexual environmental triggers because they remind you of when you would act out.

Another trigger can be an emotional trigger. Stress, anger, loneliness, and sadness can be non-sexual emotional triggers. These are the most difficult to confront. Wherever you are, at work at home, when these emotions occur you may be triggered to act out sexually. You may find yourself wanting to act out after a fight with the boss or your partner. Your mind and body are accustomed to watch porn after feeling the non-sexual emotional triggers. The same thing happens for overeaters. When they experience stress or sadness, they are inclined to binge eat. Emotions connected the behavioral addiction act with the emotion.

Understanding your triggers is critical to change sex addiction behavior. Take some time on the next page to work through your triggers.

Non-sexual Emotional Triggers

1

2

3

4

5

6

7

8

Non-sexual Environmental Triggers

1

2

3

4

5

6

7

8

Chapter Six

Family Dynamics

Approximately 1/3 of women consider porn abuse similar to an affair. Most men do not have the same concern. Men and women approach porn from different perspectives. Many women will speak to their feelings about their body, their self-esteem, their ability to become aroused, and their ability to have orgasms. Women can feel inadequate as a result of a partner's compulsive porn use which can lead to problems with sex with partner. Many men that use porn compulsively, they can become hyper-focused on the size of their genitals and whether or not they are performing properly with partner in the bedroom.

Men can get used to the type of intensity that pornography provides. Then, when they go to make love with their partner there is not that intensity and they can have trouble becoming aroused. In order to reverse the issue, a man typically needs a few months of abstaining from porn to return to normal.

There is hope. When couples seek assistance with the intention to improve their relationship, oftentimes they are able to get to the goal or at least close to their goal. Oftentimes, clinicians ask the porn addict to stop the behavior completely at least for a few months to a year.

The porn addict will need time to become re-accustomed to what normal intimate sex is like. It is not about the duration of sex and it's not about the orgasm. Intimate sex or love making is about the reconnection between partners. It is about intimacy. It involves reconnection outside of the bedroom as well. Honest communication around what is needed by both partners can be very beneficial during the time of recovery and onward. Addressing what might need attention outside of the bedroom will also likely help a great deal to reconnect partners.

Someone who is an addict will often externalize the problem. The addict may blame others around them. For example, I work so hard for my children so I need an escape. Another example would be an addict blaming the spouse for not being sexual enough or not providing enough attention. An alcoholic who gets a DUI will say things like "I shouldn't have driven the red car" and blame outside circumstances instead of themselves. Similarly, a porn addict will sometimes blame others and circumstances instead of taking responsibility for their own behavior.

Some spouses have the misconception that if they were giving their partner more sex that the partner would not have needed to turn to porn. However, when someone is addicted to a substance or a behavior, the couple could be having varied sex and constant sex, and the porn addict would likely still not able to stop the behavior. Rebuilding trust takes seeing the recovered partner in a different light. When a spouse or partner sees them as wanting recovery not only for the spouse but for themselves it is transformative for the relationship.

It is not recommended that a spouse or partner live with an addict unless they are willing to seek treatment. A spouse or partner has an important role in a sex addict's recovery because they have special leverage to get a sex addict into treatment and insist they continue their recovery process. Everyone who believes they have a problem needs to find someone to be accountable to and talk about their problems such as a therapist, coach, counselor, or support group. It is not recommended that the addict process the problems around sex addiction with a spouse. There are certified sex addiction therapists that can help as well as support groups for porn/sex addicts as well as for their spouses. It is recommended that the spouse seek their own therapy, the addict seek their own therapy, and that they also have a sex addiction specialist for couples therapy.

The spouse may be in the state of trauma for a while (typically a year or two years) depending on the severity of the betrayal. When spouses become intimate again, they can become triggered. They can be reactive, resentful, and even rageful. Spouses and partners need time to grieve. They don't need to be "calmed down." There is no need to blame the spouse for the porn addict's behavior. The spouses do not do well if they are asked to look at their part especially in the beginning (approximately the first nine months) after discovering the porn addiction behaviors. They do not need to be diagnosed with their own conditions for up to a year or more after discovering their partner's betrayal.

Spouses need time to heal. They need direction around self-care and communication. They need validation of their reality. Betrayed spouses do well in group therapy. "Betrayed Women" groups are available. They are less inclined to take out their anger on their recovering spouse and more likely to process the anger in the group therapy setting.

It is helpful if the partner or spouse takes the initiative of making an appointment with a therapist who specifically specializes in sex addiction. You can find these therapists on psychologytoday.com and search sex addiction specialists on that site.

Partners and spouses must understand that the addict's behavior is not their fault. The addict is broken and needs help. In addition, the spouse or partner needs counseling and support as much as the addict because they must process the feelings around betrayal. A spouse or partner receiving support benefits the sex addict in that the anger can be released within the support group or counseling instead of it being released on the addict.

Part III

Action Plan for Recovery

Chapter Seven

Breaking Free with Evidence-Based Tools

The first step after deciding to change is to figure out what are the unhealthy behaviors that you will stop.

Problem Behavior I Will Abstain From

_____

_____

_____

_____

_____

_____

_____

_____

_____

_____

_____

_____

_____

_____

_____

_____

_____

Now that you have listed and agreed upon the behaviors you will abstain from, it's critical to replace those behaviors with life-affirming activities and purpose.

Techniques to Kick the Habit:

1. Change your identity-Change the way you look at yourself in relation to the porn addiction habit. For instance, someone who wants to go to the gym may not actually go until they start seeing themselves as a gym-goer. They go to the store and purchase workout clothes, they throw the clothes on, and their identity has shifted enough to actually match the behavior with the new identity. One way to change identity is to see porn as something you watched as an adolescent. Start to think of yourself as someone who has sex with a real-life partner. Begin to perceive porn as childish. You are now seeing yourself as someone who used to watch porn but no longer.

2. Get yourself to the point of self-pleasuring without porn. You may want to abstain from masturbating and even sex for a few months at first before attempting. However, it is up to your discretion based on your individualized circumstance.

3. Place a parental restriction on your computer and phone for which you do not have the password to undo.

4. Replace habit with new habit-Start going to the gym, or go for a hike every time you feel an urge, go outside for a run, or go to a coffee shop during times that you would usually watch porn. Many times, in porn addiction, individuals will fall away from activities they previously enjoyed. Fill out the "Activities Worksheet" and the "Go-to List" for your new habits.

Activities You Previously Enjoyed

1

2

3

4

5

6

7

Activities You Would Like to Engage in

1

2

3

4

5

6

7

Go-to List

There are some days that you will feel triggered to act out on your behaviors. Behavioral modification is a tool clinicians use to change a behavior. Behavior modification has the potential to be highly beneficial from a sex addiction standpoint. Include things like downloading music, relaxing on the sand, finding a new podcast, or riding a jet ski, or going to a concert.

5. Remind yourself of the costs-This could lead me to erectile dysfunction, this can prevent me from meeting someone, etc. This may help more with people who are analytical. Even if this is your go-to technique to kick the habit, it's important to also have a replacement behavior as previously discussed.

6. Use Affirmations-One way to change the way you think is by using positive affirmations. Affirmations are sentence-long statements that, when repeated aloud daily, change the way you think in turn altering your behavior.

Positive Affirmations

I am living a life free from sex addiction

I am no longer seeing others as sex objects

It is not easy to say no to my sexual urges

It is easy to say no to others

I have a healthy attitude towards sex

I am in control of my own life

I am becoming free of my sex addiction

I will become free of my sexual urges

I am finding myself more positive about overcoming my addiction

I am turning into someone who is in control of their own life

I will take responsibility for my own actions

I am having a positive outlook on my future

I see people as equals and not as objects

I am not ashamed any longer

My attitude towards sex is healthy

I can connect in a deeper way than ever with my partner

I am more centered now that I am free of sex addiction

My attitude towards relationships is positive

Physical Activity

The new research regarding exercise and mood encourages clinicians to do a better job of helping clients integrate exercise into their daily lives and help them to modify their physical activity regimens. Moving your muscles is exciting because you are using one of the most effective tools for reducing depression and anxiety (which are often contributors to excessive porn use). Even if you aren't currently depressed, you likely experience stress. In these situations you will experience fight-or-flight sensations (i.e. sweating and increased heart rate) that may be unpleasant. Exercise can work as a sort of exposure therapy helping you to associate the fight-or-flight symptoms (i.e. heavy perspiration and increased heart rate) with safety instead of danger. This association can help immensely in stressful times.

Exercise Log

This is your workout log. You can use this log to both plan out your workouts and to log what you have accomplished.

Monday

_____
_____
_____

Tuesday

_____
_____
_____

Wednesday

_____
_____
_____

Thursday

_____
_____
_____

Friday

_____
_____
_____

Saturday

_____

_____

_____

Sunday

_____

_____

_____

A word about cravings:

Cravings will happen. An urge in and of itself is not bad. You are not bad because you have an urge. You need to realize that you are not the message that your brain is sending. An urge is a faulty message that is sent from the brain and it has been continually fed and strengthened. People who have successfully quit addiction, stop fearing and learn to manage urges in adaptive ways.

Step outside the urge and observe the urge without judgment. You can learn to quit porn for good by simply examining the urge. Examine your physiology. Observe your heart rate, think about what you were thinking or feeling or avoiding before you had the urge. Urges are false messages. Your brain tells you that you need to give into the urge but by replacing the act of watching porn with something else you will be able to have less cravings eventually and be re-conditioned. Pornography overstimulates the reward center of the brain and the urges are a result of the conditioning. Re-condition by observing the urge, its peak, and its diminishment and then not giving into it by doing something else. Eventually, you will re-condition your brain and urges will diminish making it easier for you.

Chapter Eight

Healthy Sex Maintenance

Porn addiction is not defined by who you are with, what you are watching, what you are doing, and how often you are watching porn. We don't qualify addiction by how much you are engaging in porn or sex addiction. However, we do define porn use as an addiction if it is impairing your functioning in life (i.e. relationship problems, work problems, time with others lost, legal problems etc.).

What is drug and alcohol sobriety? Abstaining from substances. What is sobriety from sex addiction? It's not abstaining from sex for the rest of your life. Healthy sex maintenance is involved during recovery. The sexual behaviors that need to stop should be written down and agreed upon between you and your partner.

Having sex is something between two bodies. It is the mental preparation and attitude we bring to sex that makes it intimate. Intimacy is about being connected to the person. It is about truly being present with your partner. It's about being aware that this person is meaningful to me, this is the person I love, this is the person I care for, and sex springs from that caring when you are having healthy sex in recovery. Real intimacy is about being vulnerable (which is one of the most difficult things for a sex/porn addict).

Many porn addicts believe that if we have sex and then say now we have been intimate. However, in reality, we want to be intimate and make sex an expression of that intimacy. Therefore, when you are ready to have sex again, it is advised that it is with a partner with whom you are committed. Also, make sure you have done enough recovery work that you are ready to be vulnerable and present with your partner. There are many "mindfulness" activities and practices that can help you be truly present with your partner during sex. If you want to increase the connectedness and intimacy during sex, I highly suggest that you research and practice mindfulness for sexual and non-sexual activities with your partner. This practice along with individual and group therapy with sex addiction specialists is a definitive way to healthy sex maintenance as well as full recovery.

Chapter Nine

Relapse Prevention

Relapse prevention is a method of teaching recovering persons to recognize relapse warning signs and to prevent returning to unwanted and maladaptive behaviors.

We typically hear about relapse and relapse prevention as it relates to drug and alcohol recovery. However, relapse prevention is an important concept for sex addiction and recovery. Relapse is defined as the process of becoming dysfunctional in recovery, which leads to a return to acting out behaviors. Relapse episodes are usually preceded by a series of warning signs. Usually, relapse progresses from stability (or maintenance) to physical and emotional collapse to relapse into old behaviors.

To understand the warning signs, it is important to recognize the dynamic interaction between recovery and relapse processes. Recovery can be described as related processes that occur in the following ways:

- Abstinence from sex addict behaviors
- Separation from people, places, and objects that promote sexual acting out, and forming a social network that supports recovery
- Thinking rationally and engaging in positive self-talk such as affirmations
- Managing emotions in a healthy way without resorting to compulsive behavior
- Learning to alter addictive thinking patterns that create painful feelings and self-defeating behaviors

- Identifying the mistaken core beliefs about oneself, others, and/or the world

When people who have had a stable recovery begin to relapse, they simply reverse this process.

They begin to...

- Have a limiting belief that causes irrational thoughts
- Return to addictive thinking patterns that cause painful feelings
- Engage in compulsive, self-defeating behaviors as a way to avoid negative feelings
- Seek out situations involving people who act out sexually or people who trigger them to act out
- Seek out environments in which they will be triggered to act out
- Find themselves in more pain or distress, thinking less rationally, and not using coping skills
- Find themselves in a situation in which action out seems like a logical escape from their pain, discomfort, or distress

In order to avoid a full relapse in which you've gone hours, days, weeks, or even months engaging in binge eating, you can use the following tools for relapse prevention.

Reach Out-During the maintenance phase, it is imperative that you reach out to others. Since many porn addicts are used to isolating we would call this taking "opposite action." Call a supportive and positive friend or call your mentor, coach, or therapist. Attend support groups regularly and see your sex addiction specialist regularly.

Refer to Toolbox-Utilize the coping skills outlined in this book including your Go-To List and Activities for Self-Care.

Routine-Jump back into your productive routine when you fall off.

Reinforcement-Reward is a critical part of preventing a relapse. Reward yourself as often as possible. Get tickets to a concert, go on a boat ride, or take a trip. *Reward is as important as routine.* Put reward on your calendar to avoid relapse and maintain the lifestyle you want free from porn addiction.

If you relapse (meaning you return to old behaviors), it is imperative that you do not beat yourself up because that can contribute to more shame. Clinicians call a brief return to old behaviors a "lapse" rather than a full "relapse." You have to see it as a lapse and move on from it. Replace the behavior with something like calling a friend etc. Accept that the lapse or relapse happened, say to yourself that you're going to learn from the mistake, and move forward.

Conclusion

Thank you again for reading this book.

You are not alone in this addiction. Fear and anxiety of opening up about the addiction is common. Many people have taken steps into successful porn recovery. Most couples are able to heal after discovering porn addiction within the relationship. Overall, sex addiction is an emotional disorder that needs to be treated with care and compassion so that recovery can begin.

I hope this book was able to help you understand the steps necessary for successful porn addiction recovery. You are now equipped with evidence-based tools to help you understand porn addiction, cope with the addiction, recover from the addiction, and maintain healthy intimacy.

Best wishes to you.

Porn Addiction Resources

Psychologytoday.com – search sex addiction therapists

SAA

Sex Addicts Anonymous

www.saa-recovery.org

SCA

Sexual Compulsives Anonymous

www.sca-recovery.org

S.L.A.A.

Center for Healthy Sex-
www.thecenterforhealthysex.com

Check Out My Other Books

Sex Addiction Recovered: The Ultimate Guide to Stop Sex Obsessing: Science of Sex Addiction Revealed